MW01224624

Table of Contents

Introduction

The Low FODMAP diet is a diet developed to resolve the symptoms from IBS or Irritable Bowel Syndrome. The diet eliminates or limits the intake of 4 different carbohydrates, that exists in a higher or lower number in many foods. It is a scientific fact that these carbohydrates are harder for the bowel to process than other carbohydrates. The purpose of the diet is not to follow it for the rest of your life. The purpose is to find what FODMAP-groups are triggering the symptoms from IBS and then exclude them permanently from your diet. A major part of the diet consists of testing or re-introducing foods to see which foods trigger your IBS. This is the second phase of the diet and will probably last for a couple of months. But even after this phase you will be able to continue re-introduction of foods, but more about that later. The diet consists of 3 phases. The first phase lasts approximately 4-8 weeks depending on your bowels reactions. In this phase you eliminate all high FODMAP foods from your diet, and limit the intake of "yellow" foods. When you are symptomfree you can move on to phase . In this phase you start to re-introduce high FODMAP foods in your diet. You start by re-introducing one FODMAP-group at a time following a specific schedule. You do this testing to find out exactly what FODMAP groups you bowel reacts to, so you can just exclude these from your diet. In the third phase when you tested alle groups, you know which foods to exclude and you now have your personal low FODMAP diet. It is important to keep re-challenge foods in phase 3 and beyond, because you can change tolerance over time.

Definition of FODMAPs

FODMAPs are short chain carbohydrates and sugar alcohols that are poorly digested by the body. They ferment in the large intestine (bowel) during digestion, drawing in water and producing carbon dioxide, hydrogen, and methane gas that causes the intestine to expand. This causes GI symptoms such as bloating and pain that are common in disorders like IBS. FODMAPs are in some foods naturally or as additives. They include fructose (in fruits and vegetables), fructans (like fructose, found in some vegetables and grains), lactose (dairy), galactans (legumes), and polyols (artificial sweeteners). These foods are not necessarily unhealthy products. Some of them contain fructans, inulin, and galactooligosaccharides (GOS), which are healthy prebiotics that help stimulate the growth of beneficial gut bacteria. Many of them are otherwise good for you, but in certain people, eating or drinking them causes gastrointestinal symptoms. A low FODMAP diet cuts out many common products that contain certain foods. The principle behind the diet is to give the gut a chance to heal, especially if you have GI problems like IBS. People with GI disorders may use this diet as part of their treatment. This diet may be difficult to follow, and it is advisable to contact your health care professional or a dietitian to make sure that you are on the right track and getting enough dietary nutrients that you can consume.

History

It has long been known that many short-chain carbohydrates can induce abdominal symptoms that are similar to those in patients with irritable bowel syndrome (IBS). It was hypothesized that restricting the intake of all short-chain carbohydrates that are either slowly absorbed or not digested in the small intestine should be considered together because they all have similar effects on the intestine by distending the lumen. These groups of carbohydrates were called, Fermentable, Oligosaccharides, Disaccharides and Monosaccharides and Polyols

(FODMAPs), because of the lack of a known collective term. By reducing their dietary intake, it was also hypothesized that abdominal symptoms in patients with IBS would be alleviated in patients with visceral sensitivity and a low FODMAP diet was subsequently designed. Over the last 12 years, the mechanisms of action, food content of FODMAPs and efficacy of the diet, among other aspects have been intensively studied. In many parts of the world, the low FODMAP diet is now considered a front-line therapy for IBS. For a long time, patients have recognized that certain foods can trigger gastrointestinal symptoms (including wind, diarrhea, abdominal bloating, and discomfort). Recognized food "culprits" have included milk and other dairy products, legumes and pulses, cruciferous vegetables, some fruits, and grains, especially wheat and rye. Many of these foods are known as "gas-producing foods" and were recommended to be avoided in situations of excessive flatulence and bloating. However, such foods were in lists without any linking of common components. Consequently, dietary advice pertaining to such foods was haphazard and without structure.Over the last five decades, however, advances in science and technology have meant that the food components that are present in such foods that may be responsible for these effects can be recognized. Lactose, Congenital alactasia was first reported in 1959, but it was not for another 6 years before acquired hypolactasia in adults and its causal association with diarrhea was described. The use of lactose restriction became commonplace and diagnostic tests such as measurement of lactase activity in small intestinal biopsies, blood-based lactose tolerance tests, and breath hydrogen tests were developed and applied to confirm lactose malabsorption and intolerance (i.e. when symptoms developed following ingestion of a test dose of lactose). Lactose-free diets became a dietary strategy for patients with IBS, but unfortunately did not have a major impact on symptoms overall, apart from when they were in association with ingesting a load of lactose. Fructose and sorbitol, Fructose, the fruit sugar, was implicated in symptom genesis when four patients with long-standing diarrhea and colic were reported to be cured by a fructose-free diet. In 1983, a breath hydrogen test was used to demonstrate that a child with diarrhea had fructose malabsorption and was helped by dietary fructose reduction. "Fruit-juice diarrhoea" was reported in children. Polyols, Sugar alcohols such as mannitol and xylitol have long been used as sweeteners in food manufacturing, and it was in the 1960s that their ability to induce gut symptoms was well documented in the Turku sugar studies.14 The additive effects with fructose and sorbitol (they commonly exist in foods) on symptoms was first reported in 1982.

What Does Low FODMAP Mean

FODMAP is a short for the 4 carbohydrates you eliminate from your diet:

• Fermentable

• Oligosaccharides

• Disaccharides

• Monosaccharides

• And

• Polyols

All of these carbohydrates can be found in our everyday diet and therefore the best place to start getting rid of the symptoms of IBS is by make the changes in your diet. The reason these carbohydrates cause problems for people with IBS is that they can be very difficult for the body to split and digest and therefore end up undigested in the colon. This leads to the uncomfortable symptoms like gas in you stomach, stomach ache and bloating.

How to Follow the Low-FODMAP Diet

Many doctors are now routinely recommending the low-FODMAP diet to their IBS patients. This is because the diet is the first food-based treatment that has research support for effectively reducing IBS symptoms of gas, bloating, diarrhea and constipation. With good compliance and support, approximately 70 percent of IBS patients will experience significant symptom relief. The diet is a bit tricky and will require a commitment on your part to ensure that you are choosing foods consistent with the diet. Therefore you will not want to take on the diet during a time when you will be extra busy or have limited time in your schedule for food prep and packing.

Find a Trained Professional

All of the research to date on the diet indicates that the best results are achieved when you get support from a qualified dietary professional who is well-versed in the diet.2 A dietitian or health coach is important because:

• You need to make sure that you are eating a wide variety of foods to ensure that you are taking in your daily nutritional requirements.

• It will be helpful to have support as you learn to integrate the diet into your life.

• They can help you best determine which of the FODMAP types are problematic for you.

Start a Food Diary

As you work through the various phases of the diet, you will want to keep a food diary. This will help you get a better sense of the relationship between the foods that you eat and the symptoms that you experience. This step will be especially helpful as you work through the various phases of the diet. A food diary doesn't have to be anything fancy. You just want to keep track of everything you have eaten, what symptoms you are experiencing, and any other factors that might be affecting how you feel, such as stress, your menstrual cycle, etc.

Gather Your Resources

It can be very challenging to remember which foods are low in FODMAPs and which foods are high in FODMAPs and just as challenging to find the right foods to eat. Luckily, the success of the diet has spurred the development of available resources. The low-FODMAP smartphone app from the researchers at Monash University is a must-have. It can also be helpful to purchase some low-FODMAP cookbooks and frequently visit sites that have low-FODMAP recipes. The more food options you have, the more likely you will be to comply with the diet's guidelines.

Start the Elimination Phase

To start the diet, you will need to totally eliminate known high FODMAPs foods for a period of four to six weeks. This includes foods from the following FODMAP sub-groups:

• Fructans (found in some fruits, grains, nuts, and vegetables)

• Fructose (found in some fruits)

• GOS (found in beans, chickpeas, and lentils)

• Lactose (found in some dairy products)

• Polyols (found in some fruits, vegetables, and artificial sweeteners)

• What is left to eat? Plenty of delicious, nutritious things! You can eat anything you want as long as it is low in FODMAPs.

Slowly Introduce FODMAPs Back Into Your

• After you have hopefully enjoyed a significant decrease in symptoms, it is time to slowly re-introduce some foods back into your diet. For this reintroduction phase, it is recommended that you pick one FODMAP sub-group at a time to assess the effect of each group on your body.

• Your dietary professional can help you to figure out what foods you can test your sensitivity on. Plan to test each group for a week before moving onto the next group. Start with small amounts of foods so as to not cause severe symptoms.

• If you experience no symptoms in response to your challenge foods, you can slowly start to increase the quantity you are eating. If you continue to tolerate the food, then you can conclude that you are not reactive to that particular sub-group and you can continue onto the next group.

• If you experience symptoms, you can try to test a different food from within the same sub-group. If you continue to have a reaction, you should go back to the elimination diet for one week before moving on to the next sub-group.

• After you have tested all sub-groups and have been relatively symptom-free for some time, you will want to re-test small amounts of the sub-group that you were initially reactive to. Once you have a good sense of which FODMAPs you are most reactive to, you can organize your diet so as to eat predominantly low-FODMAP, with minimal consumption of high-FODMAP foods. The goal is to keep your exposure to FODMAPs in a range that does not cause you to experience symptoms.

Keep Testing Your Range of Foods

The low-FODMAP diet is not designed to be a "forever" diet. Many foods that are high in FODMAPs are also foods that can be very good for your health. There are some concerns that FODMAP restriction can have a negative impact on your gut flora. The best thing for both your overall and your digestive health is to eat as wide a variety of healthy foods that you can. There is some evidence that once you have followed the low-FODMAP diet you will improve your ability to tolerate previously troublesome foods.5 Therefore, you will want to be sure to keep re-introducing new foods into your diet at regular intervals to see if your sensitivities have changed. One helpful way is to set a reminder in your day planner or on your smartphone to go through the reintroduction phase again every three months.

Tips If You Are New To The Low FODMAP Diet
Get A Diagnosis From Your Doctor

A lot of people self diagnose with IBS and put themselves on a low FODMAP diet, but I would not do that. It is important to get a diagnosis from your doctor, also to rule out other more life-threatening illnesses.

Consult A Registered Dietitian & Low Fodmap Diet Expert

I was diagnosed with IBS in 2013, after several medical tests and immediately my GP referred me to a dietitian, who knew about the low FODMAP diet. I am very fortunate, as I live in Australia, I was able to see the dietitian free of charge as part of the management for chronic medical condition, but if I had to pay for the visit I would have still done it. Just make sure that when you book your appointment, you ask your dietitian if she/he is an expert on the low FODMAP diet.

Follow The Low Fodmap Elimination Phase

My dietitian advised me to follow a 6 weeks of elimination diet (this was back in 2013, nowadays I have heard that the elimination phase can be also as little as 2 weeks), and she also suggested to invest a few dollars on the Monash University Low FODMAP App for iPhones or for Android Smartphones. For your convenience I have put the links to the app and other products recommended here, at the end of the article in the Useful Resources section. The elimination diet seemed hard at the beginning as I had to adjust my diet and give up all the food I was used to eat every day, but within a few days I saw a great improvement in my health and that motivated me to continue. Initially it is important to take one day at the time and do not worry about Sunday lunch at your in-laws next week). Be prepared is the key, plan what you are going to eat each day, your breakfast, lunch, dinner and snacks need to be covered, otherwise you will be tempted to reach for any food you can find. Here are some tips you may want to follow if you are going to eat out, while following a strict low FODMAP elimination diet. While on the elimination diet, keep a food diary (printable food diary here), that will help to identify any food that does not agree with you, even if it's low FODMAP (we are all different after all). By following a strict low FODMAP diet, most people see an improvement within a week or so, it is worth it.

Follow The Low Fodmap Reintroduction Phase

After 6 weeks, or however long your dietitian has asked you to be on the elimination diet, it is time to reintroduce high FODMAP food, from each FODMAP FOOD GROUP (Sugar Polyols, Lactose, Fructose, Fructans, Galacto-Oligosaccharides also called GOS). After the reintroduction phase you will still need to monitor the combination of various high FODMAP food in your diet, to understand if you react to bigger amount of that food or to the combination of food from one of the FODMAP groups.

The Low Fodmap Maintenance Phase

Well done to getting through the elimination and reintroduction phases of the low FODMAP diet. Now you should have a better idea of what food or entire food group you need to eliminate or reduce, saying that an individual should challenge that food or food group again in the future, as food sensitivity may change. Ideally what you are trying to achieve is a balanced diet that your digestive system can tolerate.

List Of Low FODMAP Foods To Eat

A list of common low FODMAP foods that are good to eat on a low FODMAP diet include:

Vegetables

• Alfalfa sprouts

• Bean sprouts

• Bell pepper

• Carrot

- Green beans

- Bok choy

- Cucumber

- Lettuce

- Tomato

- Zucchini

- Bamboo shoots

- Eggplant

- Ginger

- Chives

- Olives

- Parsnips

- Potatoes

- Turnips

Fresh Fruits

- Oranges

- Grapes

- Honeydew melon

- Cantaloupe

- Banana

- Blueberries

- Grapefruit

- Kiwi

- Lemon

- Lime

- Oranges

- Strawberries

Dairy that is lactose-free, and hard cheeses, or ripened/matured cheeses including (If you are not lactose intolerant, you may not need to avoid dairy with lactose.)

- Brie

- Camembert

- Feta cheese

- Beef, pork, chicken, fish, eggs

- Avoid breadcrumbs, marinades, and sauces/gravies that may be high in FODMAPs.

- Soy products including tofu, tempeh

- Grains

- Rice

- Rice bran

- Oats

- Oat bran

- Quinoa

- Corn flour

- Sourdough spelt bread

- Gluten-free bread and pasta

Gluten is not a FODMAP, but many gluten-free products tend to be low in FODMAPs.

- Non-dairy milks

- Almond milk

- Rice milk

- Coconut milk

Drinks

- Tea and coffee (use non-dairy milk or creamers)

- Fruit juice not from concentrate

- Water

Nuts And Seeds

- Almonds

- Macadamia

- Peanuts

- Pine nuts

- Walnuts (fewer than 10-15/serving for nuts)

- Pumpkin seeds

In some cases, portion sizes make a difference as to whether a product has enough high FODMAPs to cause symptoms. For example, a serving of almonds is a good choice that is in these short chained carbohydrates, but eat more, and you could have too many.

List Of High FODMAP Foods To Avoid

Many foods considered high in FODMAPs are healthy foods otherwise, but they can cause symptoms in some people with a sensitive gut; particularly people with IBS or other bowel diseases and disorders like SIBO. A list of common foods that you should avoid (especially if you have IBS) include:

Some Vegetables

• Onions

• Garlic

• Cabbage

• Broccoli

• Cauliflower

• Snow peas

• Asparagus

• Artichokes

- Leeks

- Beetroot

- Celery

- Sweet corn

- Brussels sprouts

- Mushrooms

Fruits, Particularly Stone Fruits Like:

- Peaches

- Apricots

- Nectarines

- Plums

- Prunes

- Mangoes

- Apples

- Pears

- Watermelon

- Cherries

- Blackberries

- Dried fruits and fruit juice concentrate

- Beans and lentils

- Wheat and rye

- Breads

- Cereals

- Pastas

- Crackers

- Pizza

Dairy Products That Contain Lactose

- Milk

- Soft cheese

- Yogurt

- Ice cream

- Custard

- Pudding

- Cottage cheese

- Nuts, including cashews and pistachios

- Sweeteners and artificial sweeteners

- High fructose corn syrup

- Honey

- Agave nectar

- Sorbitol

- Xylitol

- Maltitol

- Mannitol

- Isomalt (commonly found in sugar-free gum and mints, and even cough syrups)

Drinks

- Alcohol

- Sports drink

- Coconut water

You'll Have Increased Confidence:

• With less belly bloat, your clothes will fit better and you'll feel thinner

• 54% of IBS sufferers feel self-conscious about looks

You'll Quit Toilet Mapping:

• Live your life with freedom; no longer worrying about being close to a restroom in case of an unexpected attack

• 81% of IBS sufferers avoid situations far from bathrooms

You'll Be In A Good Mood:

• Without gas and abdominal pain, you'll feel more comfortable and in better spirits

• 50% of patients on a low-FODMAP diet had major improvement of abdominal pain

You'll Climb The Corporate Ladder Faster:

• Your improved mental and physical state will lead to less sick days and more focus on getting the job done

You'll Enhance Your Love Life:

• No more dreading dates and avoiding intimacy out of fear that expelling gas or constipation will spoil the mood

• 64% of IBS sufferers have avoided having sex because of symptoms

Alleviates IBS Symptoms

The greatest known benefit of the low-FODMAP diet is the relief it provides for people with IBS.Most of the research on the diet is in relation to IBS symptoms.A 2011 study published by Monash University found that 76% of IBS patients reported their symptoms improved on a diet that restricted high-FODMAP foods.In a 2016 review, researchers analyzed more than 20 studies on the low-FODMAP diet and found it to be an effective treatment of various gastrointestinal symptoms, including those related to IBS. The low-FODMAP diet is believed to be most effective in treating functional digestive symptoms: abdominal pain, bloating (distension), constipation, diarrhea, and flatulence (gas).

May Reduce Inflammation in IBD Patients

There's currently no cure for some irritable bowel diseases, such as ulcerative colitis and Crohn's disease. However, the low-FODMAP diet was originally associated with IBD.The researchers at Monash University are still studying the link between FODMAPs and IBD.Their latest update advises IBD patients to limit their FODMAP intake.More research is needed to determine if the low-FODMAP diet is an effective treatment for IBD. Because people with IBD have varied nutritional needs, researchers don't recommend one particular diet for all IBD patients. A low-FODMAP diet may help some people with IBD, it's not guaranteed to provide relief for everyone.

Helps Identify Dietary Triggers

People with food allergies avoid those foods to prevent allergic reactions or uncomfortable symptoms.It's the same with people who identify food triggers during the low-FODMAP program. Some experts have referred to the low-FODMAP diet as a diagnostic treatment. Because the second part of the program is a gradual reintroduction of high-FODMAP foods, followers can identify which foods are more likely to yield IBS symptoms. Though the low-FODMAP diet isn't a long-term solution, a 2016 study showed the program can improve the quality of life of people with IBS.

Followers Have Many Resources

Committing to the low-FODMAP diet even for a short period can be intimidating and stressful. Fortunately, you're not alone.Your dietician or doctor will walk you through it, but you also have access to the official FODMAP app released by Monash University. There, you can read up on the program and find recipes. There are also thousands of low-FODMAP recipes online and in cookbooks.

Cons

Though the program is beneficial for your digestive health, the process isn't easy. It can be difficult to eat out at restaurants or in social situations among other cons.

Restrictive

The main reason why the low-FODMAP diet isn't recommended long-term is that it's very restrictive. Some experts even worry about followers of the diet meeting all of their nutritional requirements because of the restrictive nature of the program. This is why people on the low-FODMAP diet must follow the protocol under the guidance of a health professional. Monash University released a statement in response to some people following the diet for long periods of time. The restrictive stage of the program is only 2-6 weeks long. Researchers explained that it's important to reintroduce FODMAPs into your diet because it encourages a varied, non-restrictive diet. FODMAPs are also beneficial to the gut in moderate amounts because they encourage the growth of good bacteria.

Not a Long-Term Solution

Patients with life-affecting digestive symptoms usually seek an answer to their health problems. Unfortunately, the low-FODMAP diet isn't a cure-all or long-term solution. The elimination phase lasts for only a few weeks. During this time, many followers report fewer symptoms. Once this phase is over, some or all symptoms may reappear. The reintroduction phase is meant to identify which foods cause the most symptoms. If the low-FODMAP diet relieved some of your symptoms, it can be tempting to remain on a modified version of the diet long-term. Experts at Monash University recommend reducing your intake of high-FODMAP foods to manage symptoms but not to eliminate them to the extent of the low-FODMAP diet.

Difficult To Modify

Vegans, vegetarians and people with food allergies must take extra caution on the low-FODMAP diet. Since it's already a restrictive diet, it can be difficult for people with additional dietary restrictions to meet their needs and consume a variety of low-FODMAP foods. However, these modifications aren't impossible. Vegans and vegetarians who consume little to no animal products are advised to get their protein from other sources: tofu, tempeh, nuts, seeds, quinoa, oats, and amaranth. People with food allergies can omit certain foods: dairy, eggs, wheat, gluten, soy, nuts, fish, etc. There's also concern that people with dietary restrictions are at further risk of nutritional deficiencies on a low-FODMAP diet. Researchers emphasize the importance of consuming a variety of compliant foods during the program.

Not Recommended for Pregnant Women and Children

Many pregnant women and children suffer from digestive problems, especially constipation. When seeking treatment, many people turn to the low-FODMAP diet. However, pregnant women and children are discouraged from trying this diet. There's not enough research to support the safety and effectiveness of this restrictive diet for either group.

A diet against Irritable Bowel Syndrome (IBS)

As i mentioned previously the low FODMAP diet is a diet specifically developed for relieving IBS.It is estimated that 1 in 7 on the planet suffer from IBS to a greater or lesser degree. The frequency in the western part of the world is estimated to be higher than in development countries.It is believed that is a result of the higher intake of fat, sugar, processed foods and too few fibres that help develop Irritable Bowel Syndrome. Although this is believed there is no scientific evidence what exactly causes IBS.For those who suffer from IBS to a high degree, it can be very difficult to be attending in social events because the symptoms can be so fierce it can be hard to focus or you have to go to the bathroom a lot. Unfortunately there are no medical treatments for IBS, nor is there an operation that can relive IBS. However there are medicin that can relieve the symptoms from IBS.But the only effective treatment are through changes in the diet. For some it will be enough to make simple changes in the daily diet, but others will need more drastic and strict changes, enter the low

FODMAP diet.The only diet to relieve IBS.Besides changing your diet or starting on the low FODMAP diet you can do a lot of thing to complement the diet and help accelerate the relieve of symptoms. Amongst are thing like exercising a minimum og 30 minutes a day, it do not have to be a hard exercise, but jogging or power walking will be just fine. If you suffer from mental conditions like anxiety or stress it will be a very good to be treated for these as well, as they can worsen the symptoms.

Recipe

Vegan Tuna Salad in Collard Green Wraps
Ingredients

• 1 1/2 cups raw walnuts

• 1 cup pitted Kalamata olives

• ¼ cup seaweed or sea veggies (I used dried wakame)

• 2 celery stalks coarsely chopped

• 2 tablespoons Bubbie's relish (I used sauerkraut, since it's what I had)

• 16 collard green leaves stems removed

• 2 heirloom tomatoes thinly sliced

• 1 tablespoon fresh chopped chives optional

Instructions

• In a food processor, pulse the walnuts until mealy. Add the olives, sea veggies, and relish (or kraut). Process again until a coarse paste. (You might have to add a tablespoon or two of water to get it smooth).

• Transfer the mixture to a medium mixing bowl and fold in the chopped celery.

• Stack two collard green leaves on a work surface so that there are no holes (one lengthwise and the other widthwise). Place ¼ cup of the untuna mixture in the center, followed by a tomato slice. Sprinkle with coarse sea salt, fresh cracked pepper and the chives (if using). Fold in the bottom, followed by the sides and secure with a toothpick or bamboo skewer and serve.

Roasted Carrot-Jalapeno Salsa with Pepitas (low FODMAP)
Ingredients

- 1 pound carrots unpeeled and cut into 1/2-inch-thick matchsticks

- 1 medium jalapeno halved

- 1 tablespoon olive oil

- 1/2 teaspoon sea salt

- 1/4 teaspoon ground cumin

- 1/4 teaspoon chili powder

- 1/4 teaspoon dried oregano

- 2 tablespoons pepitas

- 2 tablespoons fresh lime juice

Instructions

- Preheat the oven to 425 degrees F.

- On a parchment-lined baking sheet, toss the carrots, jalapenos, olive oil, sea salt, cumin, chili powder, and oregano together until well combines. Arrange in an even layer on the baking sheet, making sure the jalapeno is cut-side down. Roast in the oven until the carrots are tender and caramelized, 30 minutes.

• Remove the pan from the oven and reserve the jalapenos on a cutting board. Transfer the carrots to a high powered blender or food processor. When the peppers are cool enough to touch, remove the seeds and ribs with a spoon or pairing knife and discard. Add the flesh to the carrots, along with the pepitas, lime juice, and 1/2 cup of water. Puree until smooth, adding more water as needed to reach the consistency of tomato sauce. Taste for seasoning and add more salt as necessary.

• Serve the salsa alongside tortilla chips and crudités.

Crazy Good Coconut Oil "Chocolate" Bark
Ingredients

• 1/4 cup raw hazelnuts

• 1/4 cup raw almonds

• 1/3 cup large flake dried coconut

• 1/2 cup virgin coconut oil

• 1/2 cup cocoa or cacao powder, sifted if necessary

• 1/4 cup pure maple syrup

• 1 tablespoon smooth almond butter, optional

• pinch fine sea salt

Directions

• Preheat oven to 300F. Line a 9" square pan or a small baking sheet with two pieces of parchment paper, one going each way. Set aside.

• Add hazelnuts and almonds on a baking sheet and roast in the oven for 10 minutes. Remove baking sheet and add the coconut flakes and spread out. Continue roasting the nuts and coconut flakes for another 3-4 minutes, or until the coconut is lightly golden. Watch closely to avoid burning - coconut burns fast!

• Place hazelnuts on several sheets of damp paper towel. Wrap the hazelnuts and rub them vigorously with the paper towel until the skins fall off. It's ok if some skins don't come off. Discard the skins and roughly chop the hazelnuts and almonds.

• In a medium saucepan, melt the coconut oil over low heat. Remove from heat and whisk in the cocoa (or cacao) powder, maple syrup, and almond butter (if using) until smooth. Add a pinch of sea salt to taste. Stir in half of the almonds and hazelnuts.

• With a spatula, spoon the chocolate mixture onto the prepared parchment-lined pan or sheet and smooth out until it's about 1/4-1/2 inch thick. Sprinkle on the remaining nuts and all of the coconut flakes. Place into freezer on a flat surface for about 15 minutes, until frozen solid.

• Once frozen, break apart into bark. Store in the freezer until ready to eat. I don't recommend keeping it out on the counter long because it melts fast.

Cajun Baked Sweet Potato Fries
Ingredients

• 2 large sweet potatoes (scrubbed clean // organic when possible)

• 2 Tbsp olive, avocado, or melted coconut oil

• 1/2 tsp sea salt

• 1 1/2 tsp garlic powder

• 1 1/2 tsp smoked paprika

• 1 1/2 tsp dried oregano

• 1 tsp dried thyme*

• 1/4 tsp black pepper

• 1/4 tsp cayenne pepper*

• 1 Tbsp sugar of choice (optional // (coconut + cane are best)

Instructions

• Preheat oven to 425 degrees F (218 C).

• Leave the skin on and cut sweet potatoes into thin, even match sticks with a very sharp knife.

• Transfer to two baking sheets and drizzle with olive oil. Then sprinkle with seasonings, sugar and toss.

• Transfer fries to 1 large or 2 baking sheets (or more if making a larger batch) and arrange in a single layer to ensure they crisp up.

• Bake for 15 minutes and flip/stir to cook on the other side. Bake for 10 to 15 minutes more or until brown and crispy. You'll know they're done when the edges are dark brown and crispy.

• Remove from oven and either serve as is or drizzle with a bit of maple syrup (or honey if not vegan) to offset spiciness.

• Serve plain or with your favorite dip, such as Whiskey BBQ Ketchup.

Ingredients

• 1 tablespoon olive oil

• 4 ounces shishito peppers about 20

• ½ teaspoon sumac

• ½ teaspoon sea salt

• 1 teaspoon lemon juice

Instructions

• In a large skillet, heat the olive oil. Cook the peppers over medium heat, stirring once every minute, until blistered and soft, about 4 to 6 minutes.

• Toss the peppers with the sumac, salt, and lemon juice. Serve immediately.

Spicy Smoky Kale Chips

Ingredients

• About one bunch of kale , rinsed and dried

• Olive oil

• Salt , to taste

• About 1 tablespoon of chili flakes (or to taste)

• Sprinkling of paprika or cheyenne pepper power (optional)

Directions

• Preheat oven to 350°F.

• Remove the kale leaves from their tough end and inner stems. Cut longer leaves in half or preferred bite size pieces.

• Place kale pieces in large bowl. Start by tossing in about 1 tablespoon of olive oil. The kale leaves only need to be lightly coated with oil. Too much will make the chips too limp and greasy. Only add about 1 tablespoon of olive oil at a time. Then sprinkle in sea salt and chili flakes.

• Put the kale pieces in a single layer in a baking sheet lined. You can use parchment paper if you like for easier cleaning.

• Bake for 12-14 minutes or until crisp. About 5 minutes before they are finished, you can gently toss them in the sheet pan for more even baking. They will burn easy, be aware of how they are baking.

• For more smoky or spicy flavor, lightly dust the kale chips with paprika or cheyenne pepper power.

Baba Ganoush
Ingredients

• 3 medium-sized eggplants

• 1/2 cup (130g) tahini (sesame paste)

• 1 1/4 teaspoons coarse salt

• 3 tablespoons freshly-squeezed lemon juice

• 3 cloves garlic, peeled and smashed

• 1/8 teaspoon chile powder

• 1 tablespoon olive oil

• a half bunch picked flat-leaf parsley or cilantro leaves

Direction

• Preheat the oven to 375F (190C).

42

• Prick each eggplant a few times, then char the outside of the eggplants by placing them directly on the flame of a gas burner and as the skin chars, turn them until the eggplants are uniformly-charred on the outside. (If you don't have a gas stove, you can char them under the broiler. If not, skip to the next step.)

• Place the eggplants on a baking sheet and roast in the oven for 20 to 30 minutes, until they're completely soft; you should be able to easily poke a paring knife into them and meet no resistance.

• Remove from oven and let cool.

• Split the eggplant and scrape out the pulp. Puree the pulp in a blender or food processor with the other ingredients until smooth.

• Taste, and season with additional salt and lemon juice, if necessary. Serve drizzle with olive oil, perhaps some herbs and with crackers, sliced baguette, or toasted pita chips for dipping.

Dijon Baked Chicken Fingers
Ingredients

- 3 cups gluten-free cornflakes preferably organic, non-GMO

- 1/2 teaspoon paprika

- 1/2 teaspoon sea salt

- 1 tablespoon olive oil

- 1/4 cup Dijon mustard

- 2 garlic cloves minced

- 2 eggs

- 1 pound boneless skinless chicken breast cut into strips

Instructions

- Preheat the oven to 425 degrees F. Line a baking sheet with parchment paper.

- In a small food processor, pulse the cornflakes with the salt and paprika until finely ground. Remove to a shallow bowl and drizzle in the olive oil. Whisk with a fork until the cornflake crumbs are coated and not clumping together.

- In a second bowl, beat the eggs until smooth.

- In a large mixing bowl, combine the Dijon and garlic. Add the chicken and toss until well coated.

- Working one by one, dredge the chicken in the cornflake mixture, shaking off any excess. Dip the tenders in the egg and return them to the cornflakes, pressing down until fully coated. Arrange the tenders in an even layer on the baking sheet.

- Bake in the oven until golden and crispy, 15 to 20 minutes. Allow to cool slightly on the tray, then serve alongside ketchup and mustard.

Homemade Salsa Verde
Ingredients

- 1 ½ pounds tomatillos (about 12 medium), husked and rinsed

- 1 to 2 medium jalapeños, stemmed (omit for mild salsa, use 1 jalapeño for medium salsa and 2 jalapeños for hot salsa, note that spiciness will depend on heat of actual peppers used)

- ½ cup chopped white onion (about ½ medium onion)

- ¼ cup packed fresh cilantro leaves (more if you love cilantro)

- 2 tablespoons to ¼ cup lime juice (1 to 2 medium limes, juiced), to taste

- ½ to 1 teaspoon salt, to taste

- Optional variation: 1 to 2 diced avocados, for creamy avocado salsa verde

Instructions

- Preheat the broiler with a rack about 4 inches below the heat source. Place the tomatillos and jalapeño(s) on a rimmed baking sheet and broil until they're blackened in spots, about 5 minutes.

- Remove the baking sheet from the oven, carefully flip over the tomatillos and pepper(s) with tongs and broil for 4 to 6 more minutes, until the tomatillos are splotchy-black and blistered.

- Meanwhile, in a food processor or blender, combine the chopped onion, cilantro, 2 tablespoons lime juice and ½ teaspoon salt. Once the tomatillos are out of the oven, carefully transfer the hot tomatillos, pepper(s) and all of their juices into the food processor or blender.

• Pulse until the mixture is mostly smooth and no big chunks of tomatillo remain, scraping down the sides as necessary. Season to taste with additional lime juice and salt, if desired.

• The salsa will be thinner at first, but will thicken up after a few hours in the refrigerator, due to the naturally occurring pectin in the tomatillos. If you'd like to make creamy avocado salsa verde, let the salsa cool down before blending in 1 to 2 diced avocados (the more avocado, the creamier it gets).

Mean Green Matcha Pancakes with Raspberry Compote
Ingredients

• 1/2 cup unsweetened almond milk

• 1 large egg at room temperature

• 1 teaspoon vanilla extract

• 1 tablespoon coconut oil melted (plus more for greasing the pan)

- 3/4 cup gluten-free pancake mix

- 2 teaspoons matcha powder

- 1 pint raspberries

- Maple syrup

Instructions

- In a medium mixing bowl, whisk the almond milk, egg, vanilla, and coconut oil until combined. Add the pancake mix and matcha. Whisk until smooth, adding a splash or two more almond milk if the batter is too thick. You're going for the texture of a smoothie, not porridge.

- Heat a 5-inch cast iron skillet over a medium-high flame. Lightly brush the pan with coconut oil. Add 1/4 cup of batter to the pan. Cook until the pancake pulls away from the sides of the pan and begins to bubble towards the center, about 2 minutes. Flip and cook for another minute on the second side, until puffed and lightly browned. Remove to a plate and repeat with the remaining batter. You should have 6 thin pancakes in total.

- Meanwhile, place 3/4 of the raspberries in a small saucepan and cover with 1/4 cup water and 1 tablespoon maple syrup. Bring to a simmer over medium heat and cook, covered, until the berries have released their juices and begun to breakdown into a thick jam, about 5 minutes.

• Serve the pancakes drizzled with the compote, and garnished with the remaining raspberries. Serve alongside maple syrup and butter or ghee.

The Flu Busting, Immune Boosting Green Drink
Ingredients

• 1 cup baby spinach

• 1 leaf curly or lacinato kale stem removed

• 1 medium rib celery

• 1 medium cucumber peeled and roughly chopped

• inch peeled fresh ginger root

• 1 lime juiced

• Pinch sea salt

• Pinch of cayenne optional

• 2 drops oil of oregano optional

• 1 cup ice

Instructions

• In a high-powered blender, combine the spinach, kale, celery, cucumber, ginger, lime juice, sea salt, cayenne and oregano oil (if using). Add the ice and puree until the mixture is cold, frothy, and smooth. You want the consistency to be somewhere between a juice and a smoothie. Add more ice as necessary.

• Pour the drink into a pint-sized mason jar or glass and enjoy.

Tropical Ginger-Pineapple Smoothies MaderasLife in Nicaragua

Ingredients

• ½ cup pineapple chunks fresh or frozen

• ½ cup peeled and diced seedless cucumber

• ¼ inch peeled fresh ginger

• ¼ cup fresh mint

• 3/4 cup coconut water

Instructions

- In a food processor or blender, pulse the pineapple, cucumber, ginger, and mint until finely chopped. Add the coconut water and puree until very smooth. Add more coconut water if you like a thinner smoothie. Pour into glasses and garnish with sliced ginger and cucumber.

Low Sugar Hibiscus Smoothies with Ginger, Raspberries and Zucchini

Ingredients

- 1/2 cup hibiscus concentrate see note

- 1/2- inch knob of ginger peeled

- 1 small zucchini cut into 1-inch cubes (1 cup)

- 1/2 cup frozen raspberries

- 1/2 cup coconut almond, hemp or oat milk

- Bee pollen hemp seeds, and raspberries for garnish

Instructions

- Make the hibiscus concentrate if you haven't already (see note).

- In a blender bowl, combine the ginger, zucchini, raspberries, milk of choice, and hibiscus concentrate. Puree until smooth, adding more hibiscus concentrate or nut milk until you reach your desired consistency. Pour into a mason jar and garnish with bee pollen, more raspberries and hemp seeds, if you desire.

Banana-Berry Baked Oatmeal Bites
Ingredients

- 1 ripe banana

- 1 cup almond milk

- 1 large egg

- 1/3 cup pure maple syrup

- 1½ teaspoons pure vanilla extract

- 1 tablespoon coconut oil (in liquid form)

- 1 teaspoon lemon zest

- 2 teaspoons lemon juice

- 2 cups gluten-free rolled oats

- 1 teaspoon ground cinnamon

- ½ teaspoon kosher salt

- 1 teaspoon baking powder

- 1 cup fresh blueberries (or berries of your choice)

- 1 tablespoon brown sugar (optional)

Directions

- Preparing your Banana-Berry Baked Oatmeal Bites:

- Pre-heat your oven to 350 degrees. Spray a mini muffin tin with cooking spray.

- Place the banana in a large bowl and mash well with a fork. Add the almond milk, egg, maple syrup, vanilla extract, coconut oil, lemon zest and juice, and whisk until smooth and well combined.

- Add the dry ingredient to the wet ingredients and whisk to combine.

- Stir in the blueberries.

- Spoon the oatmeal mixture into the prepared mini muffin tin. Filling the wells almost to the top. You should have enough oatmeal for 20 bites.

- Bake for 20 minutes until the oatmeal has set and the tops of the bites are lightly browned.

• At this point you can simply let your bites cool, but I like to sprinkle the bites with a little brown sugar

• And then pop them under the broiler for a couple minutes until they get nicely browned and crispy on top.

• Let the bites cool in the muffin tin for 10 minutes. Serve warm OR carefully transfer them to a wire rack to cool completely and then refrigerate/freeze in an airtight container until you're ready to eat.

• I mean, let's take a moment to appreciate that top. And now the side view

Banana-Berry Baked Oatmeal Bites
Ingredients

• 1 ripe banana

• 1 cup almond milk

• 1 large egg

• 1/3 cup pure maple syrup

• 1½ teaspoons pure vanilla extract

• 1 tablespoon coconut oil (in liquid form)

- 1 teaspoon lemon zest

- 2 teaspoons lemon juice

- 2 cups gluten-free rolled oats

- 1 teaspoon ground cinnamon

- ½ teaspoon kosher salt

- 1 teaspoon baking powder

- 1 cup fresh blueberries (or berries of your choice)

- 1 tablespoon brown sugar (optional)

Instructions

- Pre-heat your oven to 350 degrees. Spray a mini muffin tin with cooking spray.

- Place the banana in a large bowl and mash well with a fork. Add the almond milk, egg, maple syrup, vanilla extract, coconut oil, lemon zest and juice, and whisk until smooth and well combined. In a separate bowl, combine the oats, cinnamon, salt and baking powder. Add the dry ingredient to the wet ingredients and whisk to combine. Stir in the blueberries.

• Spoon the oatmeal mixture into the prepared mini muffin tin. Filling the wells almost to the top. You should have enough oatmeal for 20 bites.

• Bake for 18-20 minutes until the oatmeal has set and the tops of the bites are lightly browned. (At this point you can simply let your bites cool, but I like to sprinkle the bites with a little brown sugar and then pop them under the broiler for a couple minutes until they get nicely browned and crispy on top.)

• Let the bites cool in the muffin tin for 10 minutes. Serve warm OR carefully transfer them to a wire rack to cool completely and then refrigerate/freeze in an airtight container until you're ready to eat.

Simple Grain-Free Granola
Ingredients

• 1/2 cup unsweetened coconut flake

• 2 cups slivered raw almonds (slivered almonds do best here)

• 1 1/4 cup raw pecans

• 1 cup raw walnuts

- 3 Tbsp chia seeds

- 1 Tbsp flaxseed meal

- 1 1/2 tsp ground cinnamon (optional)

- 2 Tbsp coconut, cane, or muscavado sugar

- 1/4 tsp sea salt

- 3 Tbsp coconut or olive oil

- 1/3 scant cup maple syrup (or sub agave or honey if not vegan)

- 1/4 cup dried blueberries (optional // or other dried fruit)

- 1/4 cup roasted unsalted sunflower seeds (optional)

Instructions

- Preheat oven to 325 degrees F (162 C) and position a rack in the center of the oven.

- In a large mixing bowl, combine the coconut, nuts, chia seeds, flax seed, cinnamon, coconut sugar, and salt.

- In a small saucepan over low heat, warm the coconut oil and maple syrup and pour over the dry ingredients and mix well.

• Spread the mixture evenly onto a large baking sheet (may require two depending on size) and bake for 20 minutes. Then remove from oven, add dried blueberries and roasted sunflower seeds, and stir.

• Increase heat to 340 degrees F (171 C) and return to oven for another 5-8 minutes, or until deep golden brown.

• The coconut oil will help this granola crisp up nicely, but be sure to watch it carefully as it browns quickly.

• Once the granola is visibly browned and done cooking (about 27 minutes total for me), remove from the oven and let cool completely.

• Store in a container with an air-tight seal, and it should keep for a few weeks.

Green Almond Milk Smoothie with Banana and Spinach
Ingredients

• 2 cups Almond Breeze Unsweetened Original Almondmilk

• 1 large banana

• 1 1/2 cups packed spinach leaves

• 1/2 cup almond butter

Instructions

• Combine all the ingredients in a blender.Puree until smooth, adding more almond milk as necessary.The consistency would be pretty thin (think fribble versus milkshake). Serve in mason jars or glasses with a straw.

Carrot Ginger Dressing

Ingredients

• 2 medium carrots peeled

• 2 inches fresh ginger peeled

• 1 small shallot

• 2 tablespoons rice vinegar

• 1 tablespoon gluten-free tamari

• 1 teaspoon sesame oil

• 1 teaspoon raw honey

• 1/4 cup cold pressed canola or safflower oil

• 1/4 cup water

- 1/2 teaspoon sea salt

Instructions

- Combine all the ingredients in a small food processor or blender. Puree until smooth. Add more water as necessary to get a smooth texture. - See more at

Arugula Pumpkin Seed Pesto
Ingredients

- ¼ cup pepitas

- 1 large garlic clove

- 4 cups baby arugula

- 2 teaspoons lemon juice

Instructions

- Combine the pepitas, garlic, arugula, lemon juice, 1/3 cup olive oil, and 1/4 teaspoon salt in a food processor or blender and puree until smooth. Add more oil as necessary. Taste for seasoning. Serve with pasta or as a condiment for fish or chicken.

The Simplest Romesco Sauce
Ingredients

- ½ pound roasted red peppers

- ¼ cup blanched whole almonds

- 1 garlic clove

- 1 tablespoon sherry or red wine vinegar

- ¼ – ½ cup olive oil

- ½ teaspoon salt

- 1/4 teaspoon red pepper flakes

Instructions

- In a small food processor, pulse the peppers, nuts, and garlic until finely chopped. Add the vinegar and puree.

- Stream in the olive oil and puree until smooth. Season with the salt and red pepper. Give it one more pulse. Serve or store in the fridge for up to two weeks.

Low FODMAP Frittata
Ingredients

- 2 handful fresh spinach

- 8 eggs

• 2 slices of prosciutto or ham

• 6 cherry tomatoes

• oil for frying

Instructions

• Wilt your spinach in a pan and put to one side.

• Crack 8 eggs into a jug and beat together.

• Tear your prosciutto into pieces and add to your jug.

• Add your spinach to the jug and mix once more.

• Season with a little salt and pepper.

• Pour into a preheated frying pan with a little oil and allow to cook for about 5 minutes on a medium heat.

• Your frittata should start to look a little cooked around the edges but still be pretty uncooked on top. At this point place your frittata in a preheated grill for another 5 minutes or until completely cooked on top.

• Remove from the grill and slice into pieces in the pan.

• You can eat this hot or cold. If you are going to eat it immediately, serve it up alongside any accompaniments.

Otherwise allow it to go cold and keep it in the fridge (When I am meal prepping I put slices ready in tupperware boxes for the week ahead).

Quinoa Berry Breakfast Bake

Ingredients

- 1 tsp butter/oil for greasing pan

- 1.5 cup quinoa dry/uncooked

- 1.5 cups strawberries

- 1 cup blueberries

- 1/2 cup raspberries

- 1/4 cup walnuts chopped (or more)

- 3 eggs

- 3 cups lactose-free milk

- 1/4 cup maple syrup or brown sugar

- 1 tbsp cinnamon

- 1 tsp ginger

- Low fodmap quinoa berry breakfast bake

Instructions

• Preheat your oven to 375 degrees F.

• Grease a large baking dish with butter or oil. Pour the quinoa into the dish and lightly shake to distribute the quinoa evenly.

• Slice the strawberries. Sprinkle the berries and walnuts over the quinoa in the dish.

• In a large bowl whisk the eggs. Stir the milk, syrup and spices into the eggs. Gently pour over the quinoa mixture.

• Bake in preheated oven for 1 hour until the quinoa has absorbed all of the liquid. Extra servings can be kept in the fridge for up to 5 days or the freezer for months.

Super Simple Roasted Carrot Soup!
Ingredients

• 6-8 large carrots

• 3 tablespoons extra virgin olive oil

• 3 cups organic chicken bone broth (substitute vegetable broth for vegan)

• 1 piece ginger (1/2 inch long piece, peeled

- 1 sprig of thyme or 1/4 tsp. dried

- 1/2 tsp dSSried chives (substitute 1/2 onion chopped)

- 1 stem organic celery, chopped into 2-inch pieces

- Salt and freshly ground pepper to taste

- 1/4 tsp ground cinnamon

Instructions

- Preheat oven to 375 degrees F.

- Peel and slice carrots into 3-inch pieces. Set on a baking sheet pan, sprinkle with about 2 tablespoons olive oil. Season with salt and pepper. Place in oven for 45 minutes to 1 hour until roasted and fork tender. Then set aside to cool.

- While the carrots are roasting, place 1 tablespoon olive oil in a pot/soup pot on medium-low heat. Place the chopped celery in the pot and cook and stir for about 5 minutes until celery is translucent. Add the thyme, ginger, chives (or onion), and cinnamon (optional) and cook for another minute.

- Add the organic chicken bone broth (recipe for homemade on this site) to the celery mixture and bring to a simmer for 5-10 minutes. Add the cooked carrots.

- Blend: either use an immersion blender right in the soup pot or use a quality blender.* Blend until creamy and desired consistency. Add more stock or water as needed. Garnish with chopped chives, chopped nuts, a swirl of non-dairy milk.

- Pour back into saucepan and heat on low until ready to serve.

No Mayo Potato Salad With Herbed Bacon & Eggs
Ingredients

- 1 1/2 pound New Potatoes or red potatoes, , washed and scrubbed

- 1/2 teaspoon salt

- 5 eggs

- 1/2 cup fresh parsley leaves, , minced

- 1/2 cup chopped fresh chives

- 1/4 cup chopped green onions (green parts only for low FODMAP)

- 6 slices bacon strips, cooked & crumbled

Mustard Vinaigrette

- 1/2 cup | 120 ml olive oil

- 3 tablespoons | 45 ml wine vinegar

- 1 1/2 teaspoon whole grain mustard

- salt to taste

Instructions

- Cut the potatoes in half and out them in a pot with just enough water to cover them. Add a pinch of salt and bring the water to a boil, then reduce down to a simmer. Cook the potatoes for about 15 minutes or until tender, but not mushy. Drain the potatoes, and rinse with cold water.

- While the potatoes are boiling add the eggs to another pot. Arrange them at the bottom in a single layer. Cover with an inch of cold water. Turn the heat to high and bring to a boil. Once the water has reached a rolling boil, turn off the heat, cover the pot and let the eggs sit in the hot water for 10-12 minutes.

• Drain the water and run the eggs under cold water to keep them from cooking further. When you're ready, peel the eggs & cut into quarters.

• To make the vinaigrette add all of the ingredients to a jar, cover and shake to combine.

• Toss the potatoes with parsley, chives, green onions, eggs, and bacon. Add the vinaigrette until the potatoes are coated. You will not need all of the dressing. Taste and season with more salt & black pepper as needed.

• You can serve as is or refrigerated it until needed up to a day.

Meatballs with Fresh Basil And Parmesan
Ingredients

• 1 lb ground beef

• 1 lb ground pork

• 3 eggs, beaten

- 2 cups gluten-free bread crumbs, plain (I like 4C Crumbs brand)

- 2 Tbsp fresh basil, chopped

- 1 tsp dried oregano

- 1 tsp crushed dried rosemary

- 1 Tbsp salt

- 2 tsp black pepper

- ½ cup aged parmesan cheese, finely grated

- 2 tsp garlic-infused oil

Instructions

- Heat oven to 400°F and prepare a baking sheet with a large piece of foil.

- Combine all ingredients except for the garlic-infused oil in a large bowl. Gently fold the ingredients into each other with your hands, but be careful not to over-mix. Stop once things are mostly incorporated. If you'd like, fry off a small piece in your skillet and check that everything is seasoned to your liking. Form the meat mixture into balls one-inch to one-and-a-half inch in diameter.

• Heat a large non-stick skillet over medium high heat. Add the garlic-infused olive oil and allow it to heat up. Brown the meatballs in the skillet in batches, about 2 minutes on each side.You aren't cooking them through, just getting a nice sear on the outside.You can skip this step if you'd like, and in that case just add another 5-8 minutes to your oven time.

• Transfer the meatballs to the foil-lined baking sheet. Cook in the oven for 10-12 minutes, then flip all the meatballs and cook for another 10-12 minutes.Test for doneness with a meat thermometer (they should be at 160°F when cooked) or cut one open to check.

• Serve My Favorite Meatballs plain, covered with marinara sauce, over spaghetti, in buns as a sandwich, or however else you desire

Low Fodmap Thai Pra Ram Tofu
Ingredients

• 1 (16 oz.) package extra firm tofu, cut in half lengthwise

• 2 Tbsp. garlic-infused olive oil, divided

• ½ cup peanut butter

- ¼ cup rice vinegar

- 2 Tbsp. reduced sodium tamari

- 1 Tbsp. maple syrup

- ½ tsp. crushed red pepper flakes

- ¼ to ½ tsp. fish sauce, optional

- 2 cups spinach

- 1 cup canned coconut milk

- Freshly chopped cilantro

Instructions

- Wrap tofu in a clean towel. Place a heavy object (like a cast iron skillet) on top of tofu for 20 minutes to press out extra moisture. Unwrap and cut pressed tofu into ½-inch cubes.

- Heat 1 Tbsp. olive oil in a large pan over medium-high heat. Add tofu, without crowding, and cook, turning occasionally, until tofu is golden brown.

- While tofu is cooking, whisk together remaining 1 Tbsp. olive oil, peanut butter, rice vinegar, soy sauce, maple syrup, crushed red pepper flakes, and optional fish sauce. Pour over tofu and stir to mix.

• Reduce heat to medium-low. Add spinach and coconut milk. Continue to cook until spinach is wilted and everything is hot, about 5 minutes. Garnish with cilantro and serve warm.

Conclusion

The low FODMAP diet it is not a long term diet, once you have gone through the process of elimination and reintroduction you should be able to consume the high FODMAP food that you can tolerate and is not causing you IBS symptoms. It is important to understand what you can or cannot eat as some high FODMAP food, such as food containing prebiotics (chicory root, raw sauerkraut, asparagus, Jerusalem artichokes, etc.) are very important as they help the good bacteria in your gut to replenish. A FODMAP modified diet has been shown to improve IBS symptoms. With careful planning this diet can be nutritionally complete. Significant improvement in the quality of life for those suffering from IBS may promote diet compliance. Gastroenterologists should refer patients with IBS to a RDN for nutrition assessment, education, and diet planning.

Made in the USA
Coppell, TX
19 February 2021

50504062R00046